HOW TO BE *Sexy*
WITHOUT LOOKING *Sleazy*

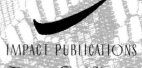

IMPACT PUBLICATIONS
Manassas Park, Virginia

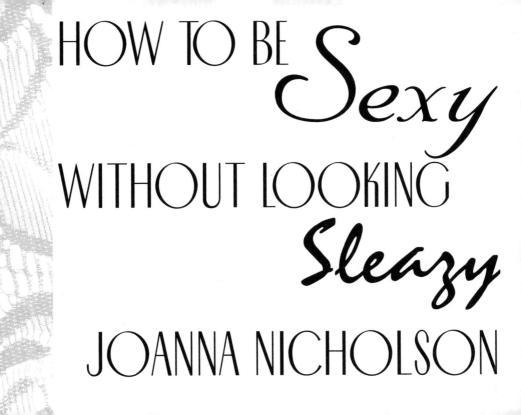

HOW TO BE *Sexy*

WITHOUT LOOKING *Sleazy*

JOANNA NICHOLSON

How to Be Sexy Without Looking Sleazy

ISBN 1-57023-013-7

Library of Congress Catalog Number 94-076585

For information on distribution or quantity discount rate,
Tel. 703/361-7300, Fax 703/335-9486, or write to:
Sales Department, Impact Publications, 9104-N Manassas Drive,
Manassas Park, VA 22111. Distributed to the trade by
National Book Network, 4720 Boston Way, Suite A,
Lanham, MD 20706, Tel. 301/459-8696.

With great appreciation to all of the sexy men and women from around the world who contributed their titillating and intimate thoughts to help make this a gem of a little book, especially to the awesome #1.

Special loving thanks:

To the "spicy" Phyllis, who continues to prove how appealing a good sense of humor is and that sexy, like a good friendship and good bottle of red wine only improves with age.

To the provocative Ceci, whose vivid and dramatic thoughts, adjectives and friendship made this book much more seductive and fun to write—may her arresting "X-factor" delightfully disrupt her entire life!

And to my incredible mother, who continues to teach by example what it means to love "nearly" unconditionally and who has proven that there really are "princes" out there who will love and cherish you even if they don't find you until you are in your seventies!

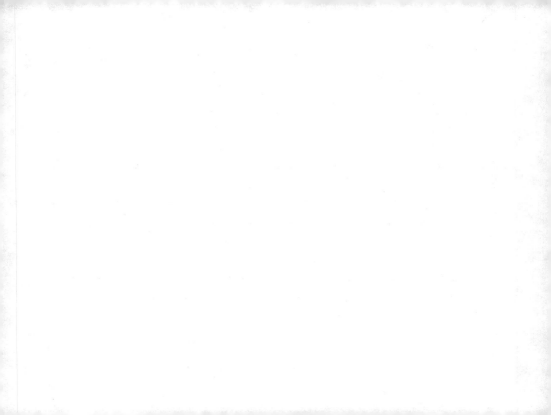

Women from every walk of life, in every age group, of every size and shape, married or single, want to be sexier. I know because I have asked them, "If you could have any look you wanted, what would it be?" Ninety-five percent answer, "Sexier!"

Their quest is threatened by the fear that they will appear foolish or sleazy. In their minds, there is a fine line between being sexy and being sleazy and they don't want to cross it — rightly so! Given the choice, they would stay "securely" mundane-looking rather than run the risk of embarrassing themselves or their men.

Yes, the differences between sexy women and sleazy women are many — how you project yourself, how you dress, how you apply your makeup, your demeanor, your attitude, a look in your eyes, the look on your face, how you move, and your body language.

I've worked with, and interviewed, women and men from all corners of the world on "How to be Sexy without Looking Sleazy." I know YOU CAN BECOME SEXIER with the right tools and attitude. Here are some of my favorite suggestions, and experiences. Get started on your sexier look by checking your Sexy I.Q.

WHAT'S YOUR SEXY I.Q.?
True or False

1. *A young woman is sexier than an older woman.* ____

2. *To be sexier, you should always have at least a little bit of skin showing.* ____

3. *A man would rather have sex with a sleazy woman than just dinner and a goodnight kiss with a sexy woman.* ___

4. *Only a sleazy woman would talk "naughty" to her man.* ____

5. *A slimmer woman is sexier than a full-figured woman.* ____

6. *To be sexy you have to be at least a little "flashy."* ____

7. *Men expect sexy women to wear quite a lot of makeup.* ____

8. *A sexy woman would not tell her man "no."* ____

9. *At work, a sexy woman should hide her "femininity."* ____

10. *To please her man, a sexy woman would fake an orgasm.* ____

11. *Cotton panties are never sexy.* ____

12. *There is a big difference between being sexy and being sleazy.* ____

13. *A sexy woman lets her man know that other men find her sexy, too.* ____

14. *To a man, a sexy woman is sexier in a bikini than she is in her glasses.* ____

15. *Sexy is a "look" more than it is an "attitude."* ____

ARE YOU RIGHT? ANSWERS IN BACK.

HOW TO BE *Sexy*
WITHOUT LOOKING *Sleazy*

Sexy and sleazy are like
Beauty and the Beast—
both are in the eye of the beholder.

A sexy woman is one that a man wants to make endless stories with…a sleazy woman is one to just "pass" his "moment" with.

Remember, sexy does not have a price-tag — there are sleazy or dowdy-looking women who have money and sexy-looking women who are on a very tight budget. Train your eye to select quality <u>looking</u> garments and accessories no matter where you shop or how much you can spend.

There is a very _fine_ line between sexy and sleazy. It's often just a matter of an inch or two: One too many buttons undone; an inch too much cleavage showing; any cleavage showing when it's not appropriate; a skirt an inch or two too short for your legs, your age, or for the occasion.

Even classy, sexy women can talk "naughty" and be risque in private. Behind closed doors anything that a consenting couple does is sexy—even "sleaze." Ask your man what words turn him on. What fantasy "outfits" does he picture you wearing — a garter belt with stockings and high heels, a G-string, or a coat and shoes with nothing else!

A sexy woman praises her man,
his body parts, brain, and humor.

Sexy women know how to pamper their men, but they also know how seductive it is to let their men pamper them. Bathe him in a bubble bath by candlelight. He will invite you to join him but "pace" it—you <u>bathe</u> him first and he will then be more than ready to bathe you!

What's irresistibly sexy to one man may be sleazy or cheap-looking to another. Find out what the type of man you want to attract finds sexy so you can appeal directly to his senses—all of them.

Sexy is sensual subtleness,
while sleazy is <u>too</u> apparent.

Some men lust after a woman who wears a tight sweater, especially if her nipples get hard. They also like tops for evening that show the uplifted bosom. Others are excited by tight pants or jeans tucked into boots. Some like skirts that are tight enough to show the shape of a woman's bottom. Sexy or sleazy? It depends on everything else about the woman.

*A man can "rent" a sleazy woman
—but would much prefer to "own"
a self-assured, sexy woman.*

Sexy women don't talk to one lover about
their other lovers — because, you see, at this
moment they don't exist for him or for you.

A man is fascinated by a sexy, accomplished woman
and _he_ feels sexier, and more confident with her at his side.

Many men find high heels sexy, but only if a woman can
walk gracefully in them. And they like sheer blouses, as long
as most of the woman's breasts are discreetly covered.

A sexy woman is always ready for the moment a man undresses her; of course, he <u>will</u> find sensuous underwear.

Sexy makeup is appropriate for the occasion and applied with a skilled hand. Overdone makeup is not sexy to the type of man you want—at least not to the type of man you want to show off to your friends.

A sexy woman likes to feel that a man's passion for her is so intense that he would move mountains to be by her side—find her, and bury himself in her bosom and ravish her (with her permission, of course)...

Sexy women do not "mother" their men.
Avoid giving advice unless asked.

Sexy women are a warm, comfortable,
loving, safe haven for their man.

A sexy woman does not use a lipliner that is
browner, or more than a hint darker, than her
lip color—match your lip liner to your lipstick
as closely as possible.

Mismatched underwear is not sexy—
neither is mundane looking cotton underwear.

Sexy women have an alluring and arousing chemistry—it is that "X" factor!! And, sexy women know how to "factor-the-X" into any scenario: a glance, a smile, a move, a word. Practice— you'll be amazed at the results!

Makeup—its magic "powders, potions, and creams" transform a woman's face, when artfully applied, into one that a man cannot take his eyes off. Getting your makeup colors and technique just right for you is a great goal, for when you accomplish this, you have an "edge" over every woman who doesn't yet know how to create a fantastic look for herself. For more details on sexy makeup looks for your bedroom, career, sports and dramatic evenings, check the Resource Section for Sexy Makeup Kits.

A sexy woman lets her man know that he excites her beyond her wildest dreams—there is no other man in her life; never has been, never will be.

Garter belts are usually found to be _classy_ on sexy women and sleazy when worn by others. They should _always_ be a surprise—and never seen by anyone other than the one man you intend to surprise.

Some women visually fulfill all of the attributes but still are not sexy. These women must learn to love men and to love to make love—not just get the technique down, but really love the entire seduction.

Bra straps that show are a major no-no. Keep bra straps in place with thread and snaps, or go without a bra if you can.

Always look a man directly in the eye. If he won't meet your gaze, you don't want him—at least not for long.

A man definitely anticipates <u>being</u> with a sexy woman— with a sleazy woman, he anticipates only HIS "release."

Have you noticed men just staring at your lips?
Yes, there are lip men! To look your most sexy, use
lipsticks in your most flattering shades of plum, fuchsia,
raspberry, red, red-coral, and coral. Also, make absolutely
certain that their brightness level is perfect for your coloring.
If you wear the wrong lipstick—too bright or too toned-down—
you can look garish or washed-out. Don't forget to coordinate
the color of your lipstick, lip pencil, blush, and nail polish
with each other, and with what you are wearing!

Sexy women stay current and contemporary-looking. Nothing is less appealing than a woman who is wearing her hair and makeup exactly as she did in high school, college, or time immemorial.

All buttoned-up can be as sexy as unbuttoned. And, all buttoned-up is much sexier than <u>too</u> unbuttoned and revealing. Before you unbutton that extra button or two, ask yourself where you are going; who's going to be there; what is your role "of the moment"; and how will others perceive you.

Some men admit to sometimes wanting sleazy women as well as sexy women—but, they also admit that it's the sexy woman that wins in the end.

Subdued self-confidence is charming and sexy.
Ungoverned self-confidence is sleazy.

Sexy women _definitely_ love sex—not just the act,
but the entire process from the first glance
to the perpetual memories.

Remove all unwanted hair from your face, nose,
underarms and legs as often as necessary—everyday,
if that's what it takes for you to feel and be sexy.

Sexy skin is beautiful, well-cared-for skin that a man cannot resist to touch. Make certain that you are taking excellent care of your skin and that the products you are using keep your skin touchable and sexy looking! If your skin feels either oily or dry, or looks "dull," the products you are using are not perfect for you. Check the Resource Section for Sexy Skin Care creams, "potions" and lotions.

Birthdays are a sleazy woman's enemy.
For the sexy woman the number
of her birthdays is irrelevant.

Some men feel that a woman who wears a ring on nearly every finger looks sleazy. Others disagree. One ring on each hand is enough. Less is more.

Sexy is not just a look, it's an "attitude." A certain behavior—an elegant, poised, self-assured behavior. Self-assurance comes from feeling good about yourself— the way you look, behave and carry yourself.

Sexy is not any one body shape or weight anymore than it is an age, hair color, or skin color. Sexy is universal.

Classy, graceful behavior is sexy.
Unclassy, ungraceful behavior is sleazy.

No safety pins, ever—even if you are certain no one is going to actually see your underwear. YOU will know the pin is there and you will behave differently.

Sexy eyes can be created with eye shadows in a variety of neutrals and colors. An unflattering color, or shadow applied in an unbecoming shape, can make you look tired, angry, over-done, swollen or old! Learn to makeup your eyes differently for a sexy bedroom look, a sexy career look, a sexy sporty look and a sexy dramatic evening look.

For public occasions, a dress shouldn't be both tight and reveal a lot of cleavage—one or the other is enough. There are rare exceptions, of course. Just make certain to err on the side of "subtle" sexiness.

A man can easily figure out if a woman is sexy
just by watching her—she doesn't have to be
wearing a mini-skirt or a low cut top.

A sexy woman will softly say, and cry out, over and over again,
her man's name during love making.

Most elegant, sexy men like women's clothing to look
very simple, perfectly pulled together, and understated
with the right combination and amount of accessories.

Develop a subtly sexy telephone voice. A lower, quieter voice sounds more intimate and will make him want to come to you, instantly. Give him _all_ of your attention—no background sounds of television or typing on the computer. And don't forget that it's as important to listen as it is to talk...

Sexy women are thrilled by both lusty quick sex and by slow, lingering sex where they can "munch" on ear lobes, lips, toes and other erogenous zones. Lengthy love making sessions do not necessarily equate to wonderful sex.

"Quality" is always better than quantity whether
we are talking about sex or clothing and accessories.
No woman whose shoes are run down,
or whose purse is falling apart, looks sexy.
Build your wardrobe around colors
that look great on you and use accessories that
coordinate with those colors in the best quality you can afford.

A sexy woman can stoop to the level of a sleazy woman but a sleazy woman can never rise to the level of a sexy woman.

A sexy woman lets her man feel that she is _his_ "private property"...if he senses that she is obviously available to other men, she isn't special enough to be with him.

When classy, sexy women go to work they are not dressed in obvious, sexy attire but neither are they dressed to deny their femininity. There is a difference. If you do not know what it is, check the Resource Section.

Naggingly demanding is not sexy. Sexy is the capability of being subtly direct and asking for what you like and want.

Scent is a most powerful tool—a major turn-on, or turn-off. Apply your fragrance sparingly everywhere you would like, or expect, his nose to be.

A sexy woman pays attention to how her man likes her to dress—if she feels good in what he prefers, and if he has good taste.

*Blush adds an astonishing glow to your face,
if you are using the right colors, and the right amount
in the right place! Avoid wearing blushes that are
too strong, too weak, too brownish, or too coral-orangy
looking for your coloring as they can make you look
garish, washed-out, muddy or sallow.*

A sexy woman takes care of all of her man's needs—his mind, heart, soul and sex. A sleazy woman fulfills only one.

Can a certain hair style look sleazy? Yes, but generally
only if it is worn by an otherwise sleazy-looking woman.
Follow the rule: elegant and simple are better;
the more dramatic the hair style, the more
simple and elegant your clothing style.

Sexy women ask their men questions like:
What do you like most? Do you like me to touch you here?
Faster? Slower? Harder? Softer? How does this feel?

It's embarrassing for a man to be with a woman who
behaves inelegantly or is dressed inappropriately—
a sexy woman would _never_ embarrass herself nor her man.

A woman can _look_ sexy until she opens her mouth.
An interesting woman is far sexier than a woman who has
a great body and no brains. Read. Listen. Continue to learn
new things. Keep up-to-date. Be a sexy renaissance woman!!

Men are attracted to sexy looking women.
If a man doesn't find you sexy, he's only interested
in wasting your time for his benefit.

Authenticity is exceedingly sexy.

Men feel that a simple, well cut dress is much sexier
than a dress that's "too" overdone.

Many men are uncomfortable with excesses and are put-off by too much jewelry, too much makeup, too much fragrance, and too much skin showing. A sexy woman discovers what her man finds appealing and dresses to please both herself and him.

Sexy women don't fake orgasms. If you aren't having them, read some books that teach you how to bring yourself to orgasm or meet with a sex therapist. Then, it will be easier for you to show your lover how to give you the pleasure you deserve. If he won't co-operate, or "rise" to your occasion, find a new lover who thinks that simply giving you pleasure is HIS greatest pleasure.

Your handshake says a lot about you. Your "presence" and carriage during the greeting is of equal importance. Cultivate a gently firm handshake—neither weak nor hard—while looking directly into his eyes.

A slip that shows in the slit of your skirt is **NOT** *sexy. If your skirt needs a slip, find a slip with a slit and position it in line with the slit in your skirt.*

Push-up bras—all bras, for that matter—and many bustiers are to be surprises for private romantic encounters. A little peek of a camisole, bustier or body suit is wonderfully enticing—more so than showing "everything."

Sexy women don't answer the phone when they are making love—turn the bell off and turn the answering machine on with the sound down so that neither of you can hear who's leaving a message.

Sexy women learn to flirt and
to play the game of seduction. Flirting
can be as simple as a special glance or
a passing smile, or as brave as a wink,
or as outrageous as sending 25 cents
(for a phone call) and your business
card over with the maitre d'…!

If your underwear is a color, it needs to be of the finest quality.
Less expensive black underwear can pass as more expensive
looking than white, beige, or colors—matching sets, of course.

Some sexy women are shy and may not be as easy
to recognize as a more outgoing sexy woman. Both types
of women are wonderful because the _right_ man is capable
of recognizing that which is not obvious to others.

Knowledge gives you attitude and carriage which IS everything! A woman who knows and feels she is sexy acts and projects sexy and classy. If you are uncertain, it can show. Make a list of those things you feel uncertain about and go to work on getting the knowledge needed to cross them off your list.

Men find the look of a woman's lips to be a powerful aphrodisiac. Learn to line your lips to give them a beautiful shape—use a lip liner and lipstick that are closely matched, and, _most_ importantly, a _delicious_ color for you!

Sexy women really, really, like themselves.
If you don't, start focusing on all of your best physical
traits and personality characteristics—in other words,
your positives. At the same time, start working on those
things you would like to change about yourself. Get better,
and better, and better, and believe me, it gets easier, and
easier until you get to the point where you are proud
and excited about who you are and the way you look.

Always wear underwear that
you would love to be caught in!
Throw out all of the rest—
there is no place for them
in your new sexy life!

If _you_ know that you're sexy, but no one else recognizes it, you need to become more memorable. Work to develop a "style" (comfortable for you) that turns heads. Focus on a great hairstyle, beautiful makeup and outfits, for work and play, that make you feel and look fabulous.

A sexy woman tells her man over and over that "HE" _is_ sexy. Compliments are golden: your hair is so soft; you smell so good; your hands are so strong—flattery and praise. Keep them simple and truthful.

Jackets and dresses that are cut to show the curves
of your body are sexy, so are some unstructured styles.
The magic, or key, is how you feel in the outfit. Remember
it's both the package and how it's wrapped that are important.

A sexy woman sleeps in, and makes love on, clean sheets.
And her surroundings are neat and clean. A candle can
hide a thousand flaws, but the morning light can bring a fright.

The amount and heaviness of a woman's eyeliner
is one of those fine lines (no pun intended) between
sexy and sleazy. If your coloring is delicate looking,
what you may think of as being a "little" can look
like a lot. If your coloring is stronger looking,
you can use more because it looks like "less" on you.

Remember to <u>feel</u> sexy all of the time,
not just on special occasions.

A sexy woman's feet are well groomed—
her toe nails are perfectly polished, never chipped—
always ready to be sucked or nibbled.

A jacket without anything under it can be sexy. If it shows
too much cleavage, add a lacy or silky camisole or bodysuit.

If your past lovers call you every once in a while,
you'll know that they found you sexy—that you are
still on their mind and perhaps even vivid in their fantasies.

Sexy women know how to dress in an appropriate way for the occasion. If you aren't absolutely sure that you look great at least 99% of the time, take classes to upgrade and update your knowledge. Check the Resource Section.

When you are naked, your face should be the same color as the rest of you! Make sure your makeup base matches the color of your neck exactly. Try a dot of the base on your neck and check the color in natural daylight.

Consider captivating underwear an investment in your future—you never know whom you may meet. And, just as your mother taught you, you never know when you might be in an accident. Wouldn't you just die if the doctor was gorgeous and you had a safety pin in your bra?

A sleazy woman may leave a man sexually satisfied but with an emptiness inside that only a sexy woman can fill.

Dress every day, night and day, exactly the way you would like to look if your favorite movie star appeared at your front door or if you ran into your ex-husband with his new girl friend or his current wife.

Sexy women use an eyebrow pencil that matches their eyebrows exactly—never one that is redder! Many women have a couple of eyebrows "missing" on the outside edge; don't forget to use a very sharp pencil to draw them in.

A sexy woman is skilled at placing a condom on her man. She can make it an erotic or playful act, depending on the mood of the moment.

Elegant, sexy men understand that, for a woman, part of being sexy is dressing, and feeling, "fashionable." Fashionable is a synonym for stylish, chic, smart, elegant, contemporary, and appropriately attired.

A sexy woman always lets her man feel that he is the smartest; that he is her best lover _ever;_ and that she has no one else in her life—but she never gives him the idea that she is his slave.

Sexy women know exquisite manners and always use them. Table manners, business manners, how to be the perfect hostess and how to be the perfect guest are examples of necessary skills that can be acquired. If you lack assurance on any level, study and/or take classes until you feel totally confident.

Sexy women discover what makes their man feel fiery and what makes him quiver with pleasure. Experiment. Watch his eyes. Experiment. Listen to his breathing rate. Experiment. Listen to him, "feel" him. Tune-in to him.

If you wear cotton panties, make sure that the cut (french cut or bikini, for example) is sensuous. Remember, sexy is in the eye of the beholder. There are men that find sporty women sexy, just as there are women that love men who enjoy sports. That doesn't mean we find their dingy white briefs sexy.

It's sexier to smell like soap than reek of perfume.
Too much of any kind of fragrance, anywhere, can
elicit a variety of thoughts—she's easy; she just doesn't
know any better; she's desperate to attract attention.

Sexy women have a marvelous sense of humor.
Heaven knows it's needed.

Completely fresh and clean body, hair, and breath is
the only way to be sexy. Unbathed, unwashed, and
unfresh is always a turn-off to any man a woman
who is reading this book would want.

Simple, feminine-looking shoes are sexy. And most men find
slim heels, not clunky heels, sexy. Make certain that you move
gracefully in them or they will have the opposite effect.

Your sexy sounds of "lovemaking" will delight your man.
He will know that he is doing what makes you feel fantastic.
The "sounds of lovemaking," if you practice expressing them,
will come naturally. If you are worried someone can hear you,
keep your sounds at "whisper" level.

Be aware of your body language and what it's saying about you.
Your posture, how you sit, stand, walk, move your hands, is all
part of your visual-package and sends a <u>very</u> strong message—
make sure you are sending the one you want.

Sometimes a sexy woman
hasn't developed her image
and is in need of polishing.

A sexy woman may meet a man's gaze across a room,
but her demeanor and expression leaves him uncertain
that she could be his. There is a subtle line between
showing interest, which can be flattering, and being too direct,
which can be a turn-off.

Make a rule when adding to your wardrobe:
I won't buy it unless it is equal to, or better than, the best look
I have right now. Follow the same rule about men.

A sexy woman doesn't worry about a man's ability to perform. She knows that she can, and will, create a wonderful memory for them both. Study books that "show and tell" you about the techniques of love-making.

Sexy women love to make love in all types of lighting, from bright revealing sunlight to pitch black, where you have the unexpected pleasure of developing an even sharper sense of touch. Arranging particularly sensual lighting often requires dimmers and the use soft pastel bulbs.

A bra that is so tight that it makes bulges above or below it is most definitely not sexy! A bra should be one of your best friends—it supports you from below, not from the straps. You should be able to let the straps fall without your breasts falling. Ask for a fitter's assistance in the lingerie department.

Understatement is always preferred to overkill.

Since first impressions are so long lasting
and so difficult to undo, use the following
guideline before you go out the door:
If you meet the man of your dreams today
and he is with his mother, would he want
her to meet you?

To undress a sexy woman takes a long, and most pleasurable, time. To undress a sleazy woman, only a few seconds. And do realize that this is in no proportion as to how much clothing she is wearing…!

Simplicity can be extremely sexy—
not to be confused with boring.

Sexy women maintain a sense of privacy, particularly
when it comes to bathroom habits. It's just not sexy
to see your lover on the toilet.

Almost every woman who is still breathing
wants to be found sexy by the "right" man.

There are a lot of sexy women that men NEVER
notice because they look washed-out. These women
are wearing clothing and makeup colors that
do not enhance their own unique coloring.
Could this be you? Check the Resource Section.

Sexy women carry on interesting conversations—
a sleazy woman isn't expected to. So, keep up-to-date
on current local and world affairs. Make an effort to read
a daily newspaper and listen to the news.

When making love a sexy woman
gives her man her full
and <u>undivided</u> attention.

*Men want to fall asleep with, and wake up beside,
a sexy woman. When they are with a sleazy woman,
they just want to "do it" and get out.*

*Sexy behavior doesn't need to lead to sex—
sometimes it is as intriguing and satisfying to know that
it could, and possibly will, in the future.*

A sexy woman is wonderfully and masterfully naughty behind closed doors. As the door opens her naughtiness adjusts accordingly.

Make certain that you taste _good_ everywhere— especially anywhere a man's lips and tongue may venture. Again, everywhere!

A sexy woman never wears curlers to bed.

Your voice is as much your signature as your fragrance. If cultivated, it can be a major turn-on—or a major turn-off if it is harsh or if you use it too much. Find the perfect balance. Record your own voice and your laugh. If you do not like what you hear, lower your voice if it sounds high; if you talk rapidly, slow down your rate of speech. Consider a voice coach.

A sexy woman is as sexy in glasses
as she is in a bikini.

Sexy women find sexy men tempting, but sexy women don't feel the need to always act on their temptations—they know that their arousing thoughts are sometimes better than a "forgettable" seduction.

A sexy woman is patient and understanding "the first time"—she knows that his strong attraction to her may cause temporary "jitters." Tell him how sexy he is — how much he excites you. Hold him. Caress him.

*For a sexy woman, seduction of her mind can be
as arousing as seduction of her body.*

*Sexy women never get drunk and most certainly
do not appreciate drunk men!*

*A sexy woman knows how to touch herself
and can show her man how she likes to be touched.*

*Too little or no makeup is not sexy most of the time.
Unless you look lovely without makeup, the only time
a totally bare face is sexy is when you're very young
or when you've just stepped out of the shower. If you
don't know how to achieve an elegant, sexy makeup look,
check the Resource Section.*

A man would rather have dinner and an engaging conversation and just a goodnight kiss with an elegant, sexy woman than have quick sex with a sleazy woman.

A sexy woman may privately tell her man, beforehand, what she has planned for him. Tell him on the way to dinner or a party; whisper in his ear at the party. Or tell him the morning before. Anticipation is an aphrodisiac.

Can women look sexy at work? Sexy women can because they know how to be subtle and how to dress appropriately for their business! Read _110 Mistakes Working Women Make and How to Avoid Them: Dressing Smart in the '90s_.

Sexy women find kissing, touching, and being touched incredibly thrilling. Kiss him everywhere. Touch him everywhere. Take note of his favorite places.

Sexy women exude sex appeal. They know that they have an indelible effect on men and they thoroughly enjoy it!

A sleazy woman drinks a lot; a classy, sexy woman who enjoys a drink, drinks a small amount of something that is _good_ quality.

Hands can be magnificent and eloquent tools.
A sexy woman always has beautifully groomed nails and
hands—and she knows how, and when, to use them.
Set aside one entire week to observe and practice the
"movement" of your hands. When you are touching a man
watch his eyes and his expression— you will soon
understand what he likes most.

*A sexy woman looks as good
from the back as she does
from the front. Always check
yourself in a full-length mirror—
from the back of your head to the floor.*

A man wants to "make" love to a sexy woman but just "do it" with a sleazy woman. A man uses a sleazy woman to attain his own quick "pleasure"; basically, a "one-man" show.

A sexy woman will let her man's imagination work. She has learned to create allure without letting all of her secrets show. And she never, ever, gives away all of her secrets at once.

A sexy woman readies her man's mind and body, subtly, a little at a time, until he feels incomparable passion. A knowing glance. Wait. A magical sexy word. Wait. A touch. Wait. A button undone. Wait...

Sexy women do not have an "agenda"—at least not one that can be detected. Sleazy women readily "promote" their availability. Many times, nothing is sexier than the unknown and/or unexpected.

If you want to look flashy, make it classy, not "crassy." If you enjoy wearing flashy clothing, make sure that it looks expensive and perfect for the occasion.

Your clothing must
always fit you well, be clean
and in good repair—
just like an ideal man.

Sexy underwear is always clean, enticing, expensive-looking and enhancing to your body style. Please do not confuse the words "expensive-looking" with the word "expensive"— as in "what it costs." Touch the fabric; if it feels scratchy or rough, it will <u>feel</u> sleazy, even if it costs a lot.

Bright colors may look fantastic on certain women and brash on others. If you don't know what's best for you, find out, now!

Sexy women are not afraid to say no to sexual turn-offs and painful or threatening activities. They would never let a man walk all over them nor undermine their self-confidence.

A sexy woman loves to touch her man everywhere and she asks him what he enjoys most. Take a class in massage— use what you learn and watch him come back for more.

Sexy women give their men
power, self-confidence, fantasies,
and dreams that last for years.
Sleazy women are a quick-fix that will
leave a man's soul hungry.

Sexy women have a self-assured walk—a great walk!
Place a full-length mirror where you can watch yourself
walk. <u>Practice</u> a graceful, sensuous walk...toes straight
ahead, legs nearly brushing each other, good, but not stiff,
posture, and gentle arm movements.

A man will happily spend time courting a sexy woman.
He may not even want to go to the effort or expense to take a
sleazy woman to dinner…just straight to bed—no frills…

Sexy women thoroughly like men —
not all men, of course, but as a "species."

Sexy women move well, with magnetic grace. Movement is not just walking and the way you use your hands—it's the way you sit down, stand up, cross your legs or move your head. Practice and observe and soon all of your movements will be sensual.

Sexy women do not "over do" their overwear nor their underwear— avoid too many frills, bows, feathers, jewels . . .

A sexy woman can have affairs for her heart, her mind, or simply for the pleasure of the sex—but whom she selects for her affairs is very important. A classy, sexy woman would never ruin her reputation for a quick thrill because she knows that her future may depend on her "past."

Sexy women are titillated by the thought of making love anywhere, and everywhere. Set intriguing "stages" for the seduction— think pillows, candles, music, sensual lighting, a favorite beverage . . .

A sexy woman knows when to say yes and when to say no.
Timing is an art.

*A totally covered up classy woman
with average looks is sexier
than a beautiful, half-naked
woman without class.*

A sexy woman knows that what one man finds arousing, another may find a turn-off, and vice versa. Treat each new man in your life as if he were your first— he is totally special and a new and unique discovery. Respond to him as you have responded to no other. You have no idea how exciting this can be—for both of you.

So, now that you know these sexy secrets…
Use them with delight! With confidence!
Discover the incomparable passion!
Experience the pleasures that only sexy women know!

Answers

1. *False. A sexy woman is sexy at any age.*

2. *False. A sexy woman is just as sexy "all covered up" as she is when she shows some skin—sometimes, more so.*

3. *False. A man that you would want would prefer the opposite.*

4. *False. In private, a sexy woman can talk as "naughty" to her man as she wants.*

5. *False. Weight, unless a woman is obese, has nothing to do with how sexy she is.*

6. *False. Subtly elegant is at least as sexy, if not more so to certain men, than being a little "flashy." If you love to look a little flashy, make sure you look elegant and are perfectly dressed for the occasion.*

7. *False. Many men find too much makeup sleazy, instead of sexy. Just the right amount of makeup for the "occasion" is sexy.*

8. *False. Sexy women are not afraid to say "no" to sexual turn-offs and painful or threatening activities.*

9. *False. Sexy women can look sexy and feminine at work because they know how to be subtle and how to dress appropriately for their business.*

10. *False. Never fake an orgasm!*

11. *False. Beautiful French cut or bikini panties made of fine cotton are sexy—especially if they are trimmed in soft lace and/or satin.*

12. *False. There is a fine line! It's often just a matter of an inch or two: one too many buttons undone; an inch too much cleavage showing; any cleavage showing when it's not appropriate; a skirt an inch or two too short for your legs, your age, or for the occasion.*

13.	*False. A sexy woman lets her man know that he excites her beyond her wildest dreams—there is no other man in her life; never has been, never will be.*

14.	*False. Good men can always recognize a sexy woman behind her glasses, and to him, she is just as sexy wearing them than when she's wearing a bikini.*

15.	*False. It is both, and even more so an attitude! You can be as sexy in jeans and a simple T-shirt as you are in a bustier—it's the way you carry yourself, the way you move, and behave, the look in your eyes, and the expression on your face.*

Resource Section

DRIVE HIM CRAZY WITH A SEXY NEW MAKEUP LOOK

Sexy 1™ Makeup *was designed to give you the most sensual look you have ever had in your life. How can it do what other makeup can't?*

It's All in The Colors! Sexy 1™ Makeup *is a division of Color 1 Associates, Inc., International Image and Style Consultants, whose makeup is used by movie stars, top models, and even Miss America!*

If Marilyn Monroe had used makeup colors that look stunning on Elizabeth Taylor, she wouldn't have looked sexy, and vice versa. If Whitney Houston were to use makeup colors that look great on Janet Jackson, she wouldn't look sexy, and vice versa.

The "secret" to your most terrific sexy look is to select the **Sexy 1 Makeup™ Kits** *that contain those colors that were specifically designed to give* <u>*your*</u> *unique coloring an incredibly sensual appearance.*

EXOTICALLY MUTED KIT
(toned-down dark colors)

Select this kit if your coloring more closely resembles that of **Kathie Lee Gifford, Sophia Loren, Whitney Houston, Raquel Welch, Wynonna, Oprah, Julia Roberts** *or* **Tina Turner**. *If you would also like to achieve a more quietly subtle look for certain sexy occasions, you may wish to add the Elegantly Gentle Kit to your "makeup wardrobe."*

ELEGANTLY GENTLE KIT
(toned-down medium/light colors)

Select this kit if your coloring more closely resembles that of **Candice Bergen, Linda Evans, Phylicia Rashad, Jane Seymour, Cybill Shepherd, Faye Dunaway** *or* **Cicely Tyson**. *If you would also like to achieve a more dramatic, yet still subtle, look for certain sexy occasions, you may wish to add the Exotically Muted Kit to your "makeup wardrobe."*

STRIKINGLY CONTRAST KIT
(bright dark colors)

Select this kit if your coloring more closely resembles that of **Elizabeth Taylor, Connie Chung, Diahann Carroll, Cher, Connie Selleca, Toni Braxton, Jaclyn Smith,** *or* **Kimberly Aiken**. *If you would also like to achieve a lighter, more delicate look for certain sexy occasions, you may wish to add the Enticingly Light & Bright Kit to your "makeup wardrobe."*

ENTICINGLY LIGHT & BRIGHT KIT
(bright medium/light colors)

Select this kit if your coloring more closely resembles that of **Marilyn Monroe, Dolly Parton, Diana Ross, Princess Di, Tyra Banks, Mary Hart** *or* **Janet Jackson**. *If you would also like to achieve a more dramatic look for certain sexy occasions, you may wish to add the Strikingly Contrast Kit to your "makeup wardrobe."*

These products are all full size, not sample size; so with the exception of perhaps your lipsticks, the products should last you at least a year.

To compliment your Sexy 1™ Makeup Kits, JoAnna has available:

Sexy 1™ Skin Care — Exceptional Products of Superior Quality at Conservative Prices

To order, call (800) 523-8496.

Joanna Nicholson personally offers classes, workshops, and seminars on total image enhancement subjects for every lifestyle, profession, and special occasion. To arrange one for your company, your organization, or for just you and your friends, call (800) 523-8496.

A SAMPLING OF PROGRAM TOPICS AVAILABLE:

How to Be Sexy Without Looking Sleazy

Discovering the Secrets of Chic Sexy Women

Trend-Setting Sexy Styles

Models' Sexy Makeup Magic Tricks

Mastering the Look of Luxury

Timeless Elegant Sexy Dressing

Sexy Anti-Aging Wardrobe, Makeup, and Hair Style Tips

How to Shop for Sexy Classy Clothing

Mastering the Art of Sexy Subtle Makeup

Appropriate Sexy Business Dressing

Or, let JoAnna design a program especially for you!

For the best advice available anywhere on your most enhancing colors, JoAnna recommends Color 1 Associates, located throughout the world. Associates offer Personal Color Charting consultations and related image services to assist you in discovering how to look great <u>all day</u>, <u>everyday</u>! Call (800) 523-8496 for the Associate nearest you.

Available soon in your local bookstore, <u>110 Mistakes Working Women Make and How to Avoid Them: Dressing Smart in the '90s</u> by JoAnna Nicholson, Impact Publications, 1995.

IMPACT RESOURCES

Impact Publications specializes in career and travel publications. For a complete annotated listing of more than 2,000 resources, contact Impact Publications. For additional copies of this book, as well as the author's professional image book for women, contact your local bookstore or complete the following form, enclose payment, and send to: IMPACT PUBLICATIONS, 9104-N Manassas Drive, Manassas Park, VA 22111-5211, Tel. 703/361-7300 or fax 703/335-9486.

Qty.   TOTAL

___ How to Be Sexy Without Looking Sleazy $6.95   _____

___ 110 Mistakes Working Women Make
     and How to Avoid Them $9.95   _____

                          SUBTOTAL   _____

                          Virginia residents include
                          4.5% sales tax   _____

                          Shipping/handling ($4.00
                          for first book and $1.00
                          for each additional book   _____